ULTIMATE DIABETIC DIET COOKBOOK FOR NEWLY DIAGNOSED 2023

A Comprehensive guide to Mastering Diabetes with Delicious and Nutritious Recipes

By

DOHERTY JONATHAN

TABLE OF CONTENT

INTRODUCTION

Are you or someone you know among the growing number of individuals recently diagnosed with diabetes? Living with diabetes can be challenging, but with the right knowledge and resources, managing the condition becomes much easier. If you're seeking a practical and comprehensive guide to help you navigate your dietary needs, we're delighted to present the ultimate solution: the Diabetic Diet Cookbook for Newly Diagnosed 2023.

Living with diabetes requires careful attention to what you eat, as diet plays a crucial role in managing blood sugar levels and overall well-being. This cookbook is specifically designed for individuals who have been recently diagnosed with diabetes, providing them with a practical and delicious approach to meal planning. Whether you're new to cooking or an experienced home chef, this cookbook is tailored to meet your dietary requirements without compromising on flavor.

Within the pages of the Ultimate Diabetic Diet Cookbook for Newly Diagnosed 2023, you'll find a wealth of expertly crafted recipes that are nutritionally balanced, diabetic-friendly, and bursting with taste. From hearty breakfasts to satisfying lunches, sumptuous dinners, and even delectable desserts, this cookbook covers it all. Every recipe is carefully created with ingredients that will help stabilize your blood sugar levels, promote weight management, and improve your overall health.

But this cookbook goes beyond just providing recipes. It's a comprehensive resource that offers valuable information about diabetes, including an overview of the condition, dietary guidelines, tips for grocery shopping, and meal planning strategies. You'll also find practical advice on portion control, food substitutions, and ways to manage cravings. With this cookbook in hand, you'll have the tools and knowledge necessary to take control of your diet and successfully manage your diabetes.

Whether you're seeking to make a positive change in your own life or supporting a loved one who is newly diagnosed, the Ultimate Diabetic Diet Cookbook for Newly Diagnosed 2023 is your go-to guide. Empower yourself with the knowledge and recipes to create delicious meals that promote a healthier lifestyle. Begin your journey to better health today with this indispensable resource, and embrace a life full of flavor and vitality while managing your diabetes effectively.

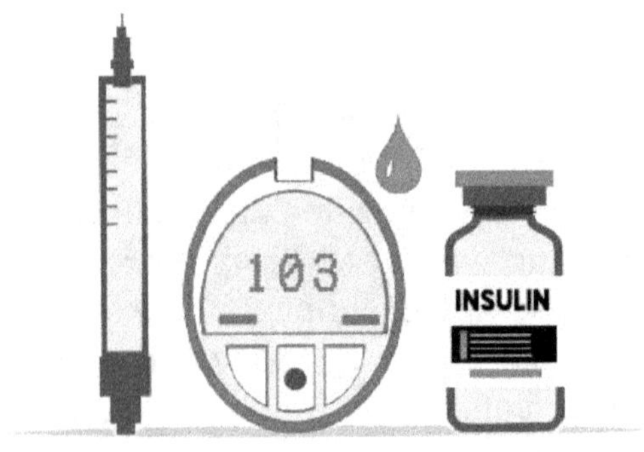

CHAPTER 1

In this chapter, we explore the fundamentals of diabetes and its impact on the body. Gain a deeper understanding of the different types of diabetes and their specific dietary considerations. Learn about the role of nutrition in managing blood sugar levels and discover practical strategies for making informed food choices that support your health and well-being.

Proper nutrition plays a crucial role in managing diabetes and promoting overall health. When it comes to diabetes, the body either does not produce enough insulin (Type 1 diabetes) or does not effectively use the insulin it produces (Type 2 diabetes). This can result in elevated blood sugar levels, which, if left uncontrolled, can lead to serious complications.

Here are key points to understand about diabetes and nutrition:

Balancing Carbohydrates: Carbohydrates must be balanced because they have the most effect on blood sugar levels. It's important to choose complex carbohydrates that are rich in fiber, such as whole grains, legumes, fruits, and vegetables. These carbohydrates are digested more slowly, leading to a more gradual rise in blood sugar levels.

Monitoring Portion Sizes: Portion control is crucial in managing diabetes. Controlling the amount of food you eat helps regulate blood sugar levels and manage body weight. It is recommended to work with a registered dietitian to determine appropriate portion sizes based on your specific needs.

Protein and Healthy Fats: Including lean protein sources, such as poultry, fish, tofu, and legumes, in your meals helps stabilize blood sugar levels and promotes satiety. Additionally, incorporating healthy fats like avocados, nuts, seeds, and olive oil can help improve insulin sensitivity and support heart health.

Glycemic Index: Based on how quickly they boost blood sugar levels, carbohydrates are ranked according to their glycemic index (GI). Foods with a low GI are digested more slowly, resulting in a more gradual increase in blood sugar levels. Including low-GI foods, such as whole grains, non-starchy vegetables, and most fruits, in your diet can help manage blood sugar levels more effectively.

Fiber-Rich Foods: Consuming adequate dietary fiber is important for individuals with diabetes. High-fiber foods, such as whole grains, legumes, fruits, and vegetables, can help regulate blood sugar levels, improve digestion, and promote a feeling of fullness.

Monitoring Sugar Intake: It's crucial to be mindful of added sugars in foods and beverages. Sugary items like sodas, candies, desserts, and processed snacks can cause blood sugar levels to spike. Opt for healthier alternatives or reduce portion sizes of sweet treats.

Individualized Approach: Every person's diabetes management plan should be tailored to their unique needs. Factors such as age, weight, activity level, and medication use should be considered when developing a personalized meal plan. Working with a registered dietitian or certified diabetes educator can help provide individualized guidance and support.

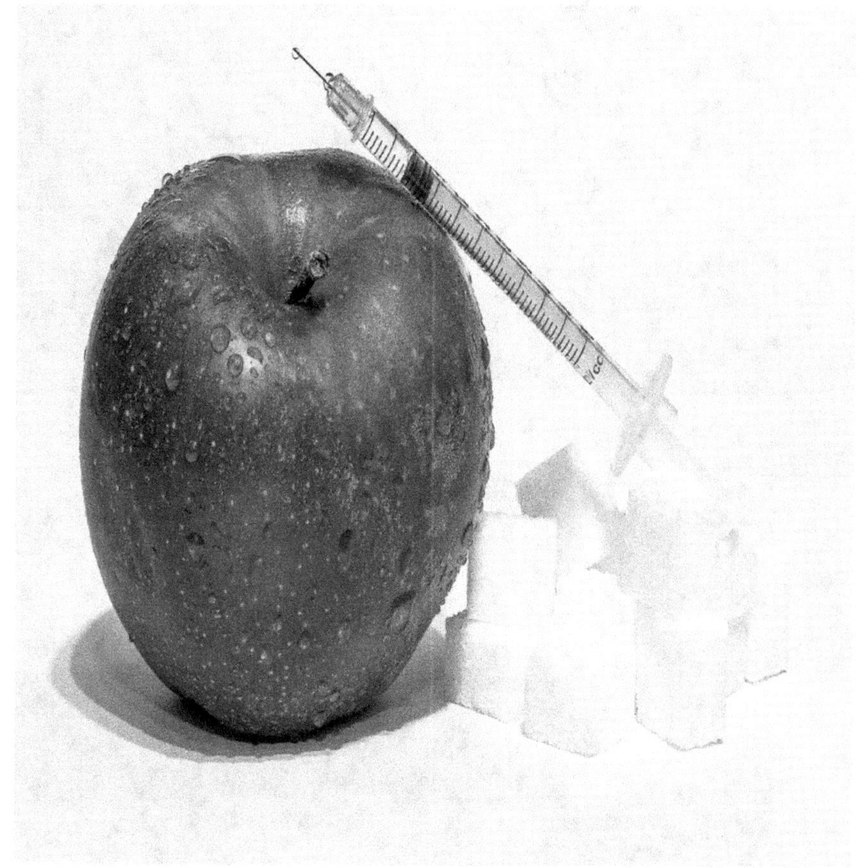

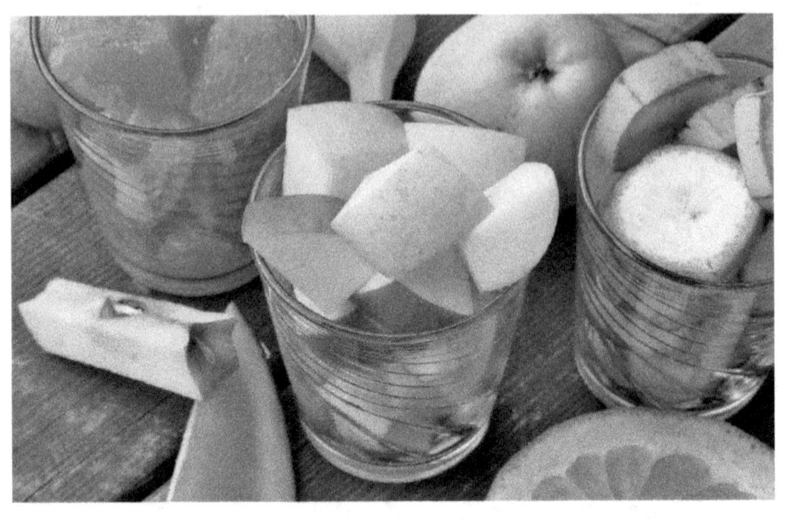

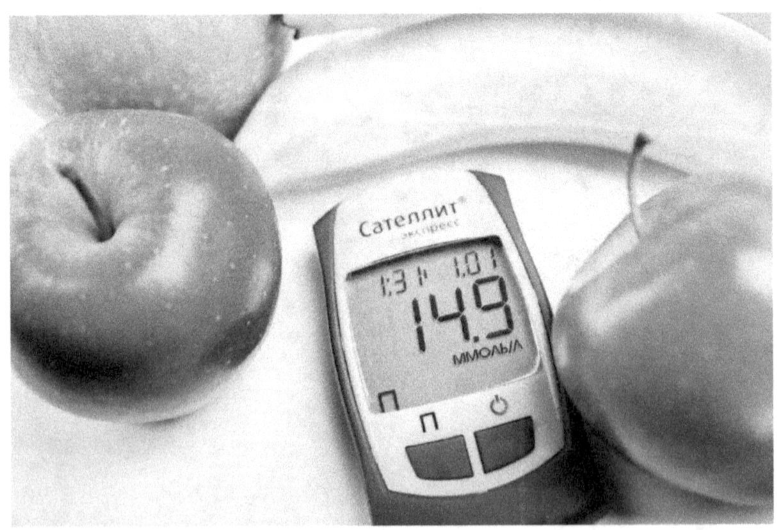
Сателлит
экспресс
1.3 1 1.01
14.9
ммоль/л
П
П

CHAPTER 2

Meal Planning and Smart Shopping

Efficient meal planning is key to maintaining a balanced diabetic diet. This chapter guides you through the process of creating personalized meal plans that align with your nutritional needs. Learn how to make smart choices at the grocery store by understanding food labels, identifying hidden sugars, and selecting diabetes-friendly ingredients. Build a well-stocked pantry and discover tips for adapting recipes to suit your preferences and dietary requirements.

Meal planning and smart shopping are essential components of maintaining a balanced and diabetes-friendly diet. This chapter will guide you through the process of creating personalized meal plans and making informed choices when grocery shopping. By incorporating these practices into your routine, you can ensure that your meals support your health goals and help manage your blood sugar levels effectively.

Understanding Meal Planning

Meal planning involves pre-determining your meals and snacks for the week, taking into consideration your nutritional needs and goals. By planning ahead, you can make healthier choices, avoid impulsive decisions, and maintain portion control. Here are some pointers to get you going:

Establish a routine: Set aside time each week to plan your meals and create a shopping list.

Consider your lifestyle: Take into account your schedule, preferences, and any dietary restrictions or food allergies.

Balance your meals: Ensure each meal includes a variety of nutrients, including lean proteins, healthy fats, whole grains, and plenty of vegetables.

Portion control: Pay attention to appropriate portion sizes to help regulate your blood sugar levels and manage your weight.

Creating a Meal Plan

A well-rounded meal plan should include a variety of foods from different food groups. Aim for a balance of carbohydrates, proteins, and fats to keep your blood sugar levels stable. Here's a step-by-step guide:

Start with breakfast: Plan nutrient-rich breakfast options such as whole grain cereals, Greek yogurt, eggs, or smoothies packed with fruits and vegetables.

Plan for lunch and dinner: Incorporate lean proteins like grilled chicken, fish, tofu, or legumes. Pair them with non-starchy vegetables and whole grains like quinoa or brown rice.

Don't forget snacks: Include healthy snacks such as raw nuts, vegetable sticks with hummus, or Greek yogurt with berries.

Hydration: Drink plenty of water all day long to stay hydrated.

Smart Shopping Tips:

Making informed choices at the grocery store is vital for a successful diabetic diet. Here's how to navigate the aisles:

Prepare a shopping list: Plan your meals in advance and create a list to guide your shopping trip. Stick to the list to avoid impulsive purchases.

Shop the perimeter: The perimeter of the grocery store typically houses fresh produce, lean proteins, and dairy products. Focus on these areas and limit your time in the processed food aisles.

Read labels carefully: Pay attention to the nutritional information, particularly carbohydrates, sugars, and serving sizes. Choose products with lower added sugars and healthier ingredient profiles.

Opt for fresh, whole foods: Choose fresh fruits, vegetables, lean meats, poultry, fish, whole grains, and low-fat dairy products. Avoid processed and sugary foods.

Stock up on pantry staples: Keep your pantry stocked with items such as whole grains, beans, nuts, seeds, and low-sodium seasonings to create healthy meals and snacks.

By incorporating meal planning and smart shopping practices into your routine, you can ensure that your pantry is filled with nutritious ingredients and that your meals align with your diabetic diet. These strategies will empower you to make mindful choices, save time and money, and support your journey toward optimal health.

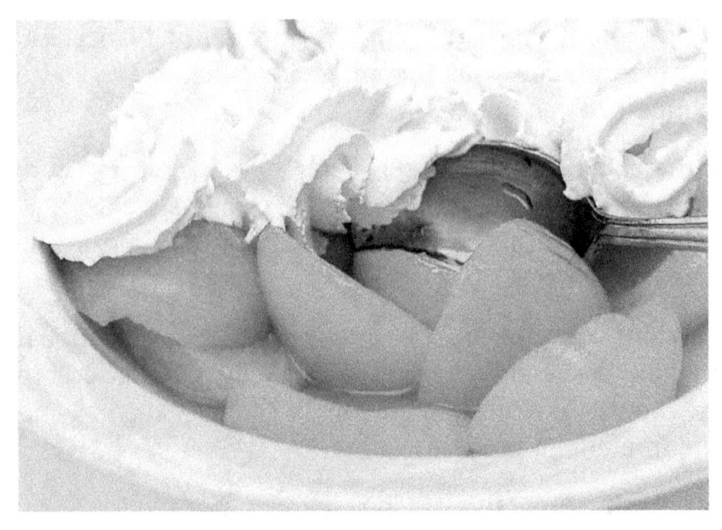

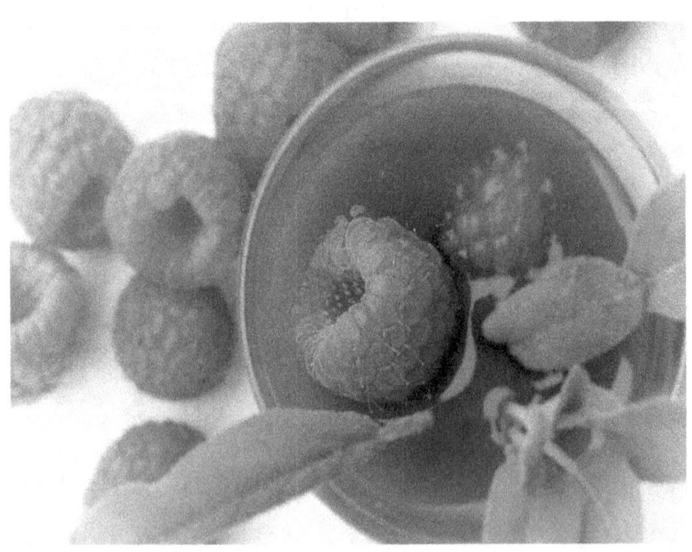

CHAPTER 3

Start your day off right with a variety of wholesome and energizing breakfast options. Explore recipes that incorporate whole grains, fiber-rich fruits, lean proteins, and healthy fats. From nutrient-packed smoothies to hearty omelets and satisfying grain bowls, these breakfast ideas will provide sustained energy and help stabilize your blood sugar levels.

Avocado Toast with Egg

Ingredients:

- 1 slice of whole grain bread
- 1/2 ripe avocado
- 1 egg
- Salt and pepper to taste
- **Optional toppings:** red pepper flakes, sliced tomatoes, or microgreens

Instructions:

1. Toasted whole grain bread can be crisped to your preferred level.
2. Mash the ripe avocado and spread it evenly on the toast.
3. In a separate pan, cook the egg to your preference (fried, poached, or scrambled).
4. On top of the avocado toast, place the cooked egg

5. Season with salt, pepper, and any optional toppings you prefer.
6. Enjoy this nutritious and satisfying breakfast.

Greek Yogurt Parfait

Ingredients:

- 1 cup Greek yogurt
- 1/4 cup granola
- 1/4 cup mixed berries (blueberries, strawberries, raspberries)
- 1 tablespoon honey or maple syrup (optional)

Instructions:

1. Greek yogurt, granola, and mixed berries should be arranged in a glass or bowl.
2. Till all the ingredients are utilized, keep layering.
3. If desired, drizzle some honey or maple syrup on top.
4. Serve chilled and savor the creamy and crunchy goodness.
5. Spinach and Mushroom Frittata

Ingredients:

- 4 large eggs
- 1 cup baby spinach leaves
- 1/2 cup sliced mushrooms
- 1/4 cup shredded cheese (such as cheddar or feta)
- Salt and pepper to taste
- 1 tablespoon olive oil

Instructions:

1. Preheat the oven to 350°F (175°C).
2. heat olive oil over medium heat, in an oven-safe skillet.
3. Add mushrooms and sauté until they start to brown.
4. Add spinach leaves and cook until wilted.
5. In a bowl, whisk the eggs and season with salt and pepper.
6. Pour the whisked eggs into the skillet, ensuring they cover the vegetables evenly.
7. Sprinkle shredded cheese on top.
8. Transfer the skillet to the preheated oven and bake for about 15 minutes or until the frittata is set.
9. Before slicing, take it out of the oven and let it cool a little.
10. Serve warm as a delicious and protein-packed breakfast.

Banana Nut Smoothie

Ingredients:

- 1 ripe banana
- 1 cup almond milk
- 2 tablespoons peanut butter or almond butter
- 1 tablespoon honey or maple syrup
- 1 tablespoon chia seeds (optional)
- Handful of ice cubes

Instructions:

1. In a blender, combine the ripe banana, almond milk, peanut butter or almond butter, honey or maple syrup, chia seeds (if using), and ice cubes.

2. Blend until smooth and creamy.
3. Pour into a glass and garnish with a sprinkle of chia seeds, if desired.
4. Sip and enjoy this refreshing and protein-rich smoothie.

Quinoa Breakfast Bowl with Berries and Almonds

Ingredients:

- 1/2 cup cooked quinoa
- 1/4 cup almond milk (or your preferred milk)
- 1/4 teaspoon vanilla extract
- 1 tablespoon honey or maple syrup
- 1/4 cup mixed berries (blueberries, strawberries, raspberries)
- 1 tablespoon sliced almonds

Instructions:

1. In a saucepan, heat the cooked quinoa with almond milk and vanilla extract over medium heat. Stir in honey or maple syrup until well combined. Cook until well heated for a few minutes.
2. Transfer the quinoa mixture to a bowl.
3. Top with mixed berries and sliced almonds.
4. Drizzle additional honey or maple syrup, if desired.
5. Enjoy this protein-packed and fiber-rich breakfast bowl.

Veggie Breakfast Burrito

Ingredients:

- 2 large eggs
- 1 whole wheat tortilla or wrap
- 1/4 cup chopped bell peppers (any color)
- 1/4 cup chopped onions1/4 cup chopped tomatoes
- Handful of spinach leaves
- Salt and pepper to taste
- 1 teaspoon olive oil

Instructions:

1. In a bowl, whisk the eggs and season with salt and pepper.
2. Over medium heat, the olive oil in the pan is warmed.
3. Sauté bell peppers, onions, tomatoes, and spinach until tender.Over the veggies in the pan, pour the whisked eggs.
4. Scramble the eggs and cook until set.
5. Warm the whole wheat tortilla or wrap in a separate pan or microwave.
6. Place the scrambled eggs and vegetable mixture onto the tortilla or wrap.
7. Roll it up, tucking in the sides.
8. Serve warm and enjoy this hearty and flavorful breakfast burrito.

Overnight Oats with Berries and Almonds

Ingredients:

- 1/2 cup rolled oats
- 1/2 cup almond milk or your preferred milk

- 1/4 cup Greek yogurt
- 1 tablespoon chia seeds
- 1 tablespoon honey or maple syrup
- 1/4 cup mixed berries (blueberries, strawberries, raspberries)
- 1 tablespoon sliced almonds

Instructions:

1. In a jar or container, combine rolled oats, almond milk, Greek yogurt, chia seeds, and honey or maple syrup.
2. Stir well to ensure the ingredients are well mixed.
3. Add mixed berries and sliced almonds on top.
4. Cover the jar or container and refrigerate overnight.
5. In the morning, give the mixture a good stir and enjoy this ready-to-eat and fiber-rich breakfast.

Green Smoothie Bowl

Ingredients:

- 1 ripe banana
- 1 cup spinach leaves
- 1/2 cup almond milk or your preferred milk
- 1 tablespoon almond butter or peanut butter
- 1 tablespoon honey or maple syrup
- Toppings: sliced fruits, granola, chia seeds

Instructions:

1. In a blender, combine the ripe banana, spinach leaves, almond milk, almond butter or peanut butter, and honey or maple syrup.
2. Blend until smooth and creamy.
3. Pour the green smoothie into a bowl.

4. Top with your favorite sliced fruits, granola, and chia seeds for added texture and nutrients.
5. Enjoy this refreshing and nutrient-packed smoothie bowl.

Egg and Veggie Muffin Cups

Ingredients:

- 6 large eggs
- 1/2 cup chopped bell peppers (any color)
- 1/4 cup chopped onions
- 1/4 cup chopped tomatoes
- Handful of spinach leaves
- Salt and pepper to taste
- Cooking spray or oil for greasing

Instructions:

1. Preheat the oven to 350°F (175°C).
2. Cooking spray or a little bit of oil should be used to grease a muffin pan.
3. In a bowl, whisk the eggs and season with salt and pepper.
4. Stir in bell peppers, onions, tomatoes, and spinach.
5. Pour the egg and vegetable mixture evenly into the greased muffin tin.
6. Bake for about 15-20 minutes or until the muffin cups are set and slightly golden.
7. Before taking them out of the tin, let them cool for a few minutes.
8. Serve warm or refrigerate for later use.
9. Enjoy these convenient and protein-packed egg and veggie muffin cups.

Peanut Butter Banana Protein Smoothie

Ingredients:

- 1 ripe banana
- 1 cup almond milk or any desired milk
- 2 tablespoons peanut butter (or almond butter)
- 1 scoop vanilla protein powder
- Handful of ice cubes

Instructions:

1. In a blender, combine the ripe banana, almond milk, peanut butter, protein powder, and ice cubes.
2. Blend until smooth and creamy.
3. Pour into a glass and enjoy this protein-rich and satisfying smoothie.
4. These energizing breakfast recipes will provide you with a nutritious and delicious start to your day. Enjoy experimenting with different flavors and ingredients to find your favorite combinations. Remember, always adapt the recipes to suit your dietary needs and preferences.

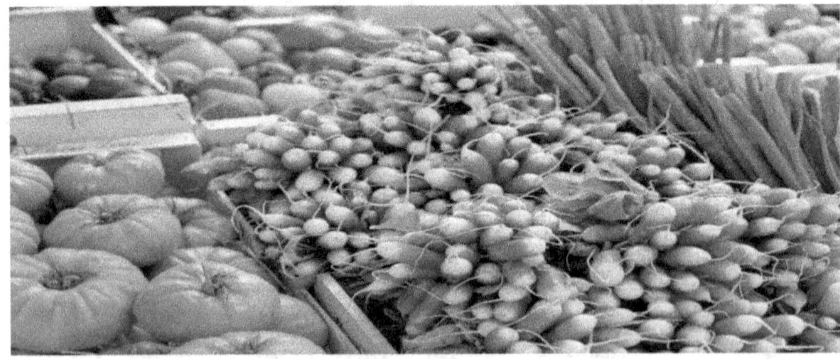

CHAPTER 4

Lifestyle Tips for Diabetes Management

Managing diabetes extends beyond the kitchen. In this chapter, we delve into strategies for incorporating physical activity into your daily routine, managing social gatherings, dining out, and traveling with diabetes. Discover tips for coping with stress, maintaining emotional well-being, and finding support through diabetes support groups and online resources.

Managing diabetes extends beyond just dietary choices. It entails changing your lifestyle to be more holistic. In this chapter, we will explore various lifestyle tips that can support your diabetes management and overall well-being. By incorporating these tips into your daily routine, you can enhance your quality of life and effectively manage your condition.

Regular Physical Activity

Engaging in regular physical activity is essential for managing diabetes. It helps lower blood sugar levels, improves insulin sensitivity, promotes weight management, and enhances overall cardiovascular health. At least 150 minutes per week of moderate-intensity aerobic activity, such as brisk walking, cycling, swimming, or dancing, should be your goal. Additionally, incorporate strength training exercises at least two days a week to build muscle and improve overall body composition.

Stress Management

Blood sugar levels might become raised as a result of ongoing stress. Therefore, it's essential to learn stress management techniques. Explore stress-reduction techniques such as deep breathing exercises, meditation, yoga, mindfulness, or engaging in hobbies and activities that bring you joy and relaxation. Creating a balance between work, personal life, and self-care is essential for overall well-being.

Regular Blood Sugar Monitoring

Monitoring your blood sugar levels regularly is important to track your progress and make informed decisions regarding your diabetes management. Work with your healthcare provider to establish a monitoring schedule and understand the target ranges for your blood sugar levels. This information can guide you in making necessary adjustments to your diet, medication, or physical activity routine.

Adequate Sleep

Getting sufficient, high-quality sleep is vital for diabetes management. Poor sleep can disrupt hormonal balance, impair insulin sensitivity, and affect overall energy levels and mood Sleep for 7-8 hours each night, uninterrupted. Establish a regular sleep routine, create a calming sleep environment, and practice good sleep hygiene habits, such as avoiding electronic devices before bed and keeping a consistent sleep schedule.

Regular Medical Check-ups

Regular visits to your healthcare provider are important for monitoring your diabetes and overall health. Schedule routine check-ups to assess your blood sugar control, adjust medications if necessary, and address any concerns or questions you may have. Additionally, stay up to date with preventive screenings, such as eye exams, cholesterol checks, and foot examinations, as they can help identify and manage potential complications of diabetes.

Diabetes Education and Support

Participating in diabetes education programs and seeking support from healthcare professionals, diabetes educators, and support groups can be highly beneficial. These resources can provide you with valuable information, self-management techniques, and a supportive community to navigate the challenges of diabetes. Stay informed about the latest research, treatment options, and lifestyle strategies to empower yourself in effectively managing your condition.

Social Support and Engagement

Surrounding yourself with a supportive network of family, friends, and loved ones can positively impact your diabetes management. Inform them about your condition, educate them about diabetes, and seek their understanding and support. Engage in social activities, hobbies, and interests that promote a sense of fulfillment and joy, as social connectedness and emotional well-being are integral parts of a healthy lifestyle.

Diabetes-Friendly Dining Out

Eating out can be challenging when managing diabetes, but with careful planning, it can still be enjoyable. Research menus in advance, choose restaurants that offer healthier options, control portion sizes, and make specific requests to accommodate your dietary needs. Be mindful of hidden sugars, choose grilled or baked options instead of fried foods, and opt for water or unsweetened beverages. Communicate with your server and don't hesitate to ask for modifications to suit your requirements.

Traveling with Diabetes

When traveling, proper preparation is key to managing your diabetes effectively. Pack all necessary medications, supplies, and snacks to avoid interruptions in your routine. Keep your insulin or medication in a cool place if needed. Research local healthcare resources at your destination and ensure you have appropriate travel insurance. Maintain a balanced diet and continue your exercise routine as much as possible while traveling.

Positive Mindset and Self-Care

Maintaining a positive mindset and practicing self-care are essential aspects of managing diabetes. Be kind to yourself, acknowledge your little wins, and concentrate on progress rather than perfection. Prioritize self-care activities that promote relaxation, joy, and overall well-being. This may include engaging in hobbies, practicing mindfulness, spending time in nature, or seeking professional counseling if needed.

CONCLUSION

Embracing a Vibrant Life with "Ultimate Diabetic Diet Cookbook for Newly Diagnosed 2023"

As you reach the conclusion of Ultimate Diabetic Cookbook for Newly Diagnosed 2023, I hope you feel empowered, inspired, and equipped to navigate your new journey with diabetes. This cookbook has been designed to support you in embracing a vibrant and fulfilling life while effectively managing your condition through delicious and diabetes-friendly meals.

Throughout these pages, you have discovered a wealth of knowledge, practical tips, and a wide array of flavorful recipes. From energizing breakfasts to hearty main courses and delectable desserts, each recipe has been thoughtfully crafted to not only meet your dietary requirements but also awaken your taste buds and bring joy to your dining table.

I encourage you to approach your new found dietary needs with curiosity and creativity. Use the recipes in this cookbook as a foundation for exploring your own culinary innovations, experimenting with flavors, and adapting dishes to suit your preferences. Remember that a diabetic-friendly diet can be both nutritious and delicious, and with the right ingredients and techniques, you can enjoy a wide range of satisfying meals.

Beyond the recipes, Ultimate Diabetic Cookbook for Newly Diagnosed 2023 has emphasized the importance of a holistic approach to diabetes management. It has provided insights into the impact of diabetes on the body, the significance of portion control, the role of physical activity, and the value of self-care and seeking support. By embracing these lifestyle changes, you can optimize your overall health and well-being.

As you continue on your journey, I encourage you to stay connected with your healthcare provider, diabetes educators, and support networks. They can provide you with ongoing guidance, answer your questions, and offer invaluable support throughout your diabetes management.

Remember that managing diabetes is a lifelong commitment, and each day presents an opportunity to make choices that support your health and vitality. Be patient with yourself, celebrate your progress, and remain open to new discoveries along the way.

Wishing you a life filled with good health, delicious meals, and the empowerment to thrive with diabetes.